Anti-Concussion Training Intermediate Field Manual for Athletes, Coaches and Parents Seeking Improved Safety.

By Steven Helmicki

Copyright 2013 Primordial Strength Inc.

ISBN: 978-1-300-61712-9

--   ------------------------------------

Name   Date

Date of Introductory Manual Phases A-E Completion: -----------------------------

Phase F- 2 weeks Perform twice weekly.

Workout 1

Primordial 4-Way Neck Machine 10lbs x 8 reps all 4 ways.

Straight Bar Shrugs 65lbs x 25 reps

Workout 2

Primordial 4 Way Neck Machine 10lbs x 10 reps all 4 ways.

Straight Bar Shrugs 75 lbs x 15 reps

Workout 3

Primordial 4 Way Neck Machine 10lbs x 12 reps all 4 ways.

Straight bar Shrugs 75lbs x 20 reps

Workout 4

Primordial 4 Way Neck Machine 10lbs x 15 reps

Straight Bar Shrugs 75lbs x 25 reps

Training Date:_____   Anti-Concussion Phase:_____

Workout Number:_____   Sport:--

Any potential concussive incidents in daily life or primary athletic activity:---
----

If you filled the above space out you should seek medical attention immediately.

Any neck/trap or head discomfort prior to training---

If you experience any discomfort you should not train and seek medical attention.

Prescribed Rehabilitation/Physical Therapy work:---

Neck/Trap
Workout_____
_____
_____
_____
_____

Training Date:_____   Anti-Concussion Phase:_____

Workout Number:_____   Sport:---

Any potential concussive incidents in daily life or primary athletic activity:---------------------------------------
----

If you filled the above space out you should seek medical attention immediately.

Any neck/trap or head discomfort prior to training--

If you experience any discomfort you should not train and seek medical attention.

Prescribed Rehabilitation/Physical Therapy work:---

Neck/Trap
Workout_____
_____
_____
_____
_____

Training Date:_____   Anti-Concussion Phase:_____

Workout Number:_____   Sport:---

Any potential concussive incidents in daily life or primary athletic activity:--
----

If you filled the above space out you should seek medical attention immediately.

Any neck/trap or head discomfort prior to training--

If you experience any discomfort you should not train and seek medical attention.

Prescribed Rehabilitation/Physical Therapy work:---

Neck/Trap
Workout_____
_____
_____
_____
_____

Training Date:_____   Anti-Concussion Phase:_____

Workout Number:_____   Sport:--

Any potential concussive incidents in daily life or primary athletic activity:--
----

If you filled the above space out you should seek medical attention immediately.

Any neck/trap or head discomfort prior to training---

If you experience any discomfort you should not train and seek medical attention.

Prescribed Rehabilitation/Physical Therapy work:--

Neck/Trap
Workout_____
_____
_____
_____
_____

Training Date:_____   Anti-Concussion Phase:_____

Workout Number:_____   Sport:--

Any potential concussive incidents in daily life or primary athletic activity:--
----

If you filled the above space out you should seek medical attention immediately.

Any neck/trap or head discomfort prior to training---

If you experience any discomfort you should not train and seek medical attention.

Prescribed Rehabilitation/Physical Therapy work:---

Neck/Trap
Workout_____
_____
_____
_____
_____

Training Date:_____   Anti-Concussion Phase:_____

Workout Number:_____   Sport:--

Any potential concussive incidents in daily life or primary athletic activity:---
----

If you filled the above space out you should seek medical attention immediately.

Any neck/trap or head discomfort prior to training--

If you experience any discomfort you should not train and seek medical attention.

Prescribed Rehabilitation/Physical Therapy work:--

Neck/Trap
Workout_____
_____
_____
_____
_____

Training Date:_____   Anti-Concussion Phase:_____

Workout Number:_____   Sport:---

Any potential concussive incidents in daily life or primary athletic activity:--------------------------------------
----

If you filled the above space out you should seek medical attention immediately.

Any neck/trap or head discomfort prior to training--

If you experience any discomfort you should not train and seek medical attention.

Prescribed Rehabilitation/Physical Therapy work:--

Neck/Trap
Workout_____
_____
_____
_____
_____

Training Date:_____   Anti-Concussion Phase:_____

Workout Number:_____   Sport:--

Any potential concussive incidents in daily life or primary athletic activity:--
----

If you filled the above space out you should seek medical attention immediately.

Any neck/trap or head discomfort prior to training--

If you experience any discomfort you should not train and seek medical attention.

Prescribed Rehabilitation/Physical Therapy work:--

Neck/Trap
Workout_____
_____
_____
_____
_____

Training Date:_____   Anti-Concussion Phase:_____

Workout Number:_____   Sport:---

Any potential concussive incidents in daily life or primary athletic activity:--
----

If you filled the above space out you should seek medical attention immediately.

Any neck/trap or head discomfort prior to training--

If you experience any discomfort you should not train and seek medical attention.

Prescribed Rehabilitation/Physical Therapy work:---

Neck/Trap
Workout_____
_____
_____
_____
_____

Phase G- 2 weeks. Perform Twice weekly.

Workout 1
Primordial 4 Way Neck Machine 15lbs x 8 reps all 4 ways
Seated Alternated Dumbbell/Kettlebell Shrugs 30lbs x 15 reps

Workout 2
Primordial 4 Way Neck Machine 15lbs x 10 reps all 4 ways
Seated Alternated Dumbbell/Kettlebell Shrugs 30lbs. x 20 reps

Workout 3
Primordial 4 Way Neck Machine 15lbs x 12 reps all 4 ways
Seated Alternated Dumbbell/Kettlebell Shrugs 30lbs. x 25 reps
Workout 4

Primordial 4 Way Neck Machine 15lbs x 15 reps all 4 Ways
Seated Alternated Dumbbell/Kettlebell Shrugs 30lbs x 30 reps

Training Date:_____   Anti-Concussion Phase:_____

Workout Number:_____   Sport:--

Any potential concussive incidents in daily life or primary athletic activity:---------------------------------------
----

If you filled the above space out you should seek medical attention immediately.

Any neck/trap or head discomfort prior to training---

If you experience any discomfort you should not train and seek medical attention.

Prescribed Rehabilitation/Physical Therapy work:---

Neck/Trap
Workout_____
_____
_____
_____
_____

Training Date:_____   Anti-Concussion Phase:_____

Workout Number:_____   Sport:---

Any potential concussive incidents in daily life or primary athletic activity:--
----

If you filled the above space out you should seek medical attention immediately.

Any neck/trap or head discomfort prior to training---

If you experience any discomfort you should not train and seek medical attention.

Prescribed Rehabilitation/Physical Therapy work:---

Neck/Trap
Workout_____
_____
_____
_____
_____

Training Date:_____   Anti-Concussion Phase:_____

Workout Number:_____   Sport:--

Any potential concussive incidents in daily life or primary athletic activity:---------------------------------------
----

If you filled the above space out you should seek medical attention immediately.

Any neck/trap or head discomfort prior to training--

If you experience any discomfort you should not train and seek medical attention.

Prescribed Rehabilitation/Physical Therapy work:---

Neck/Trap
Workout_____
_____
_____
_____
_____

Training Date:_____   Anti-Concussion Phase:_____

Workout Number:_____   Sport:---

Any potential concussive incidents in daily life or primary athletic activity:-------------------------------------
----

If you filled the above space out you should seek medical attention immediately.

Any neck/trap or head discomfort prior to training---

If you experience any discomfort you should not train and seek medical attention.

Prescribed Rehabilitation/Physical Therapy work:--

Neck/Trap
Workout_____
_____
_____
_____
_____

Training Date:_____   Anti-Concussion Phase:_____

Workout Number:_____   Sport:--

Any potential concussive incidents in daily life or primary athletic activity:------------------------------------
----

If you filled the above space out you should seek medical attention immediately.

Any neck/trap or head discomfort prior to training---

If you experience any discomfort you should not train and seek medical attention.

Prescribed Rehabilitation/Physical Therapy work:---

Neck/Trap
Workout_____
_____
_____
_____
_____

Training Date:_____   Anti-Concussion Phase:_____

Workout Number:_____   Sport:--

Any potential concussive incidents in daily life or primary athletic activity:--------------------------------------
----

If you filled the above space out you should seek medical attention immediately.

Any neck/trap or head discomfort prior to training--

If you experience any discomfort you should not train and seek medical attention.

Prescribed Rehabilitation/Physical Therapy work:---

Neck/Trap
Workout_____
_____
_____
_____
_____

Training Date:_____   Anti-Concussion Phase:_____

Workout Number:_____   Sport:---

Any potential concussive incidents in daily life or primary athletic activity:---
----

If you filled the above space out you should seek medical attention immediately.

Any neck/trap or head discomfort prior to training--

If you experience any discomfort you should not train and seek medical attention.

Prescribed Rehabilitation/Physical Therapy work:--

Neck/Trap
Workout_____
_____
_____
_____

Training Date:_____   Anti-Concussion Phase:_____

Workout Number:_____   Sport:--

Any potential concussive incidents in daily life or primary athletic activity:---------------------------------------
----

If you filled the above space out you should seek medical attention immediately.

Any neck/trap or head discomfort prior to training--

If you experience any discomfort you should not train and seek medical attention.

Prescribed Rehabilitation/Physical Therapy work:---

Neck/Trap
Workout_____
_____
_____
_____
_____

Phase H- Three weeks. Perform twice weekly.

Workout- Seated Free Hand Neck Resistance 10 reps all four Ways. Snatch Grip Barbell Shrugs 65lbs x 15 reps. Add 5 reps per week on each exercise throughout the 3 weeks.

▲ Seated Free Hand Neck Resistance
Sit on a flat bench with your back straight and head up. Place both of your hands directly on your forehead. Inhale and push your head downward in a semicircular motion as far as you comfortably can as you resist your neck muscles with your arms. At the low position, push your head upward and back in a semicircular motion as far as you comfortably can, resisting your neck muscles with your arms. Do the prescribed number of repetitions and then place both hands on the back of your head and repeat the movement. Then place the palm of your right hand on the right side of your head and resist from side to side until the prescribed number of repetitions are complete. Then change positions to the left side to finish the exercise. This movement may be performed in a standing, seated, kneeling, or lying position.

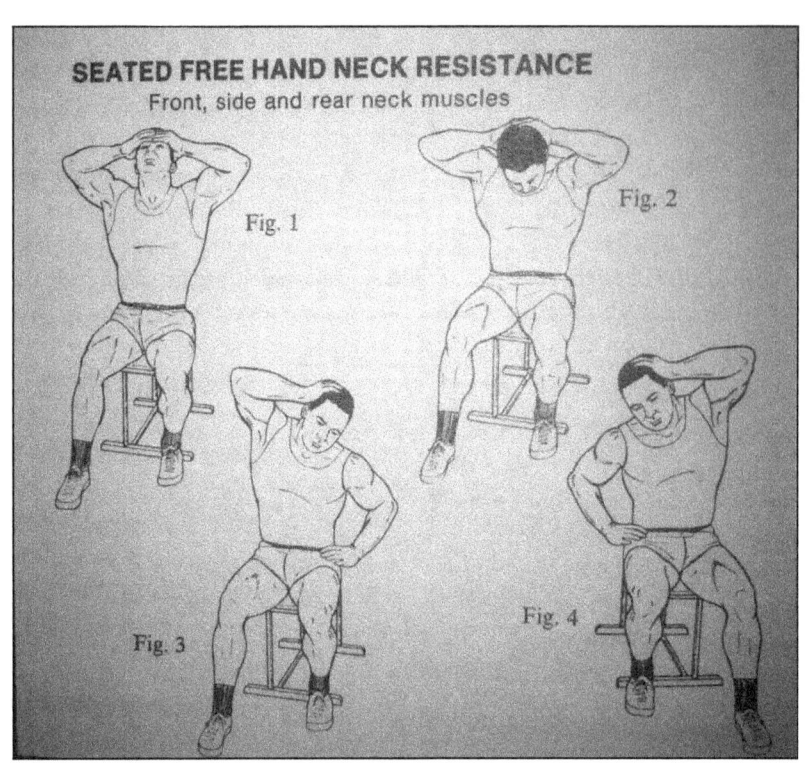

SEATED FREE HAND NECK RESISTANCE
Front, side and rear neck muscles

Fig. 1

Fig. 2

Fig. 3

Fig. 4

Training Date:_____   Anti-Concussion Phase:_____

Workout Number:_____   Sport:---

Any potential concussive incidents in daily life or primary athletic activity:-------------------------------------
----

If you filled the above space out you should seek medical attention immediately.

Any neck/trap or head discomfort prior to training--

If you experience any discomfort you should not train and seek medical attention.

Prescribed Rehabilitation/Physical Therapy work:--

Neck/Trap
Workout_____
_____
_____
_____
_____

Training Date:_____   Anti-Concussion Phase:_____

Workout Number:_____   Sport:--

Any potential concussive incidents in daily life or primary athletic activity:--
----

If you filled the above space out you should seek medical attention immediately.

Any neck/trap or head discomfort prior to training--

If you experience any discomfort you should not train and seek medical attention.

Prescribed Rehabilitation/Physical Therapy work:---

Neck/Trap
Workout_____
_____
_____
_____
_____

Training Date:_____   Anti-Concussion Phase:_____

Workout Number:_____   Sport:--

Any potential concussive incidents in daily life or primary athletic activity:------------------------------------
----

If you filled the above space out you should seek medical attention immediately.

Any neck/trap or head discomfort prior to training--

If you experience any discomfort you should not train and seek medical attention.

Prescribed Rehabilitation/Physical Therapy work:--

Neck/Trap
Workout_____
_____
_____
_____
_____

Training Date:_____   Anti-Concussion Phase:_____

Workout Number:_____   Sport:---

Any potential concussive incidents in daily life or primary athletic activity:---
----

If you filled the above space out you should seek medical attention immediately.

Any neck/trap or head discomfort prior to training--

If you experience any discomfort you should not train and seek medical attention.

Prescribed Rehabilitation/Physical Therapy work:---

Neck/Trap
Workout_____
_____
_____
_____
_____

Training Date:_____   Anti-Concussion Phase:_____

Workout Number:_____   Sport:--

Any potential concussive incidents in daily life or primary athletic activity:---
----

If you filled the above space out you should seek medical attention immediately.

Any neck/trap or head discomfort prior to training---

If you experience any discomfort you should not train and seek medical attention.

Prescribed Rehabilitation/Physical Therapy work:--

Neck/Trap
Workout_____
_____
_____
_____
_____

Training Date:_____   Anti-Concussion Phase:_____

Workout Number:_____   Sport:---

Any potential concussive incidents in daily life or primary athletic activity:---------------------------------------
----

If you filled the above space out you should seek medical attention immediately.

Any neck/trap or head discomfort prior to training---

If you experience any discomfort you should not train and seek medical attention.

Prescribed Rehabilitation/Physical Therapy work:--

Neck/Trap
Workout_____
_____
_____
_____
_____

Training Date:_____   Anti-Concussion Phase:_____

Workout Number:_____   Sport:---

Any potential concussive incidents in daily life or primary athletic activity:------------------------------------
----

If you filled the above space out you should seek medical attention immediately.

Any neck/trap or head discomfort prior to training--

If you experience any discomfort you should not train and seek medical attention.

Prescribed Rehabilitation/Physical Therapy work:--

Neck/Trap
Workout_____
_____
_____
_____
_____

Training Date:_____   Anti-Concussion Phase:_____

Workout Number:_____   Sport:--

Any potential concussive incidents in daily life or primary athletic activity:--
----

If you filled the above space out you should seek medical attention immediately.

Any neck/trap or head discomfort prior to training--

If you experience any discomfort you should not train and seek medical attention.

Prescribed Rehabilitation/Physical Therapy work:--

Neck/Trap
Workout_____
_____
_____
_____
_____

Proceed to Anti-Concussion Advanced Manual.

www.ingramcontent.com/pod-product-compliance
Lightning Source LLC
Chambersburg PA
CBHW081541280526
45788CB00010B/3319

* 9 7 8 1 3 0 0 6 1 7 1 2 9 *